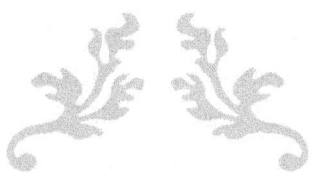

THE ULTIMATE GUIDE TO COSMETIC SURGERY MARKETING

The 7 Secrets the Top Surgeons Do Not Want You to Know About Patient Generation

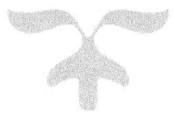

DAN WARDROPE

WWW.FLEXXDIGITAL.COM

46 Goldstone Road, Hove, BN3 3RH

Contents

I would like to dedicate this book to my wife, Emily.

"Some people can never believe in themselves, until someone believes in them."

Good Will Hunting (1997)

Housekeeping

A quick bit of housekeeping before we get going.

I use the Google URL shortener throughout this book to allow you to easily follow a recommended link without having to remember complicated URLs.

For example:

goo.gl/ccCScV

The goo.gl bit always remains the same: only the /ccCScV part needs to be remembered! Hope that makes sense.

Alright, let's get started.

Introduction:
Finding Unicorns

"In the republic of mediocrity, genius is dangerous."

Robert G. Ingersoll

The cosmetic surgery industry is growing we are told.

So why are we all still working so hard to achieve incremental advances? If you have ever had to stifle a yawn when your marketing agency reports, with a self-satisfied smile, that fractional growth in visits and enquiries are a sign that you are heading in the right direction, then this book is for you.

Why worry over such small details when there is a much bigger picture that you should be focussing on?

You haven't trained for years to watch with jealous envy the one or two practices that dominate your market claim all the accolades, get all the attention and win all the patients.

You haven't built your practice on a solid foundation in order to constantly glance over your shoulder at the cowboys and bottom dwellers that are lowering their prices and nibbling at your margins.

You deserve something more.

Don't lose sight of your original targets. Never forget your early ambitions to dominate the field.

It's time to stop looking for increments and start chasing unicorns.

In this book I'm going to show you how mediocrity is a disease that will slowly blind you and surely bind you. If you continue to market your practice in the same way that everyone else does you will only ever achieve the same results as them. You will be fighting over the scraps that fall from the table of the larger concerns.

I'm going to help you get your feet firmly under that table.

- You can command market-leading prices for your procedures.
- You can be seen as an expert in your field.
- You can win the trust and respect of your peers, your public and the press.
- You can reach more prospects and convert more of them into patients. Not just one or two more: many more.

You can change the game rather than play the game. It's not going to take years but it will take courage and vision.

Forget what the competition is doing: they are all doing the same thing anyway. You are about to do something different. You are about to learn the seven secrets of patient generation that the market leaders do not want you to know about.

Let's find those unicorns.

The Health of the Cosmetic Surgery Industry

"Plastic surgery 'booming' in the UK."

James Gallagher,

BBC News, 3 February 2014

Is your business booming or is it just ticking along?

The UK economy appears buoyant once more and new statistics from the British Association of Aesthetic Plastic Surgeons (www.baaps.org.uk) reveal that you should be experiencing double digit growth year on year.

Since 2012 not one single individual procedure has declined in popularity. In fact, every cosmetic operation has risen very significantly.

Even the PIP implant scare of June 2012 has had no adverse effect: breast surgery is up a whopping 13%.

Dr. Rajiv Grover is a consultant plastic surgeon and the president of BAAPS. He holds the responsibility for auditing the UK's cosmetic surgery industry: this is what he has to say about its robust health and future prospects.

"Both the UK economy and the British public seem to be well on the way to regaining their shape with the most impressive rise in demand for cosmetic surgery we have seen since the onset of the recession in 2008.

Patient confidence, and also consumer confidence, has returned with Britons choosing to spend on procedures with proven track records, such as liposuction which remains the gold standard for body contouring.

The continued double digit rise of cosmetic surgery underlines the fact that, whether it is breast augmentation or anti-ageing procedures like facelifting, the public are choosing tried and tested surgical methods rather than the magical-sounding quick fixes that fail to deliver promised results."

In 2013 there were 50,122 cosmetic surgical procedures carried out in the UK. This represents an impressive 16.5% increase on the previous year.

The top ten surgical procedures for both men and women were:

1.	Breast augmentation	11,135	(up 13%)
2.	Blepharoplasty (eyelid surgery)	7,808	(up 14%)
3.	Facelift/Necklift	6,380	(up 13%)
4.	Breast Reduction	5,476	(up 12.5%)
5.	Rhinoplasty	4,878	(up 17%)
6.	Liposuction	4,326	(up 41%)
7.	Abdominoplasty	3,466	(up 16%)
8.	Fat Transfer	3,302	(up 14.5%)
9.	Browlift	2,138	(up 17%)
10.	Otoplasty (ear correction)	1,213	(up 14%)

The facts and figures don't lie: if you are a cosmetic plastic surgeon in the UK there has never been a better time to grow your practice.

Such booming figures, however, do not go unnoticed.

Whether it is pop-up injectable clinics run by underqualified GPs, or dangerous package deals offered abroad, there has never been more competition.

It is the established surgeons, with reputation and celebrity status, who will continue to win the high-end patients.

Meanwhile the surgeons who slash their prices in a frantic bid to compete will win only the scarcely profitable low-end patients (until, of course, someone else undercuts them).

The future is bright indeed for those with established clinics and established credentials. If you want to join them I'm about to show you how it can be done.

And it doesn't take years.

It won't require a massive marketing budget.

But its ongoing effects on your practice will last for a very long time.

The secret of breaking into this competitive space is a perfectly planned and well-executed marketing strategy. How do I know this? Simply because I have helped many other surgeons achieve it using exactly these methods.

Let me tell you a bit about myself.

My Background

"Flexx Digital have taken cosmetic surgery marketing farther than it's ever been taken before, by providing marketing solutions so powerful that I challenge anyone to implement their methods and not quintuple their business within the first six months."

Dr. Pouria Moradi, Sydney

My name is Dan Wardrope and I am the founder and director of Flexx Digital (www.flexxdigital.com), a marketing agency that specialises in patient generation for plastic and cosmetic surgeons in the UK and Australia.

Day in and day out I see the looks of frustration, and the raised eyebrows of scepticism, on the faces of my clients when they hear the term 'marketing agency'. Many of them have worked their way fruitlessly through four or five agencies: they have been sold variations of the same poor marketing techniques over and over again.

I share their frustration.

I understand your doubts and concerns.

But I offer something very different in both approach and results: I'd like to share these secrets with you.

Let's start with the basics.

After many years of working with the industry I have noticed that there are just two types of clients who win.

One group I refer to as the bottom dwellers. These are those who aim to compete on price. Unfortunately such wins are never sustainable: all it takes is for another aggressive entrant to the market, with a lower price, to erode any gains that they have achieved.

The second group consists of the expert, or celebrity, surgeons. Gains made here last. The surgeons in question have usually worked for many years to establish themselves as an authority on a particular procedure. They have done this through a blend of experience, persistence and highly targeted marketing.

The beauty of becoming an expert is that patients start to find you. They arrive at your practice with an essential ingredient: trust.

The celebrity surgeon is blessed with some kind of 'patient attraction formula' that no amount of spend on advertising can buy.

I have tried to make 'ordinary' marketing work for an 'ordinary' practice and it's a long, hard slog. So much so that I no longer take on clients who just want me to turn the same old tired marketing tricks for them. I've found something better: something that actually works time and time again.

To be honest, I needed to discover the secret to success as much as my clients did.

I am probably the most competitive guy you will ever meet. In a past life I was a professional basketball player, and the sport's 'never say die, win at all costs' instinct has stayed with me.

I knew I needed to change the traditional marketing strategy so that surgeons, who did not want to entertain entering a price war yet didn't have the luxury of 30 years' experience under their belt, could still dominate their market.

So I went out and I did just this. And it worked.

So I did it again.

And again.

And again.

Along the way I realised that this is a formula that works every time: I could teach this stuff.

This is why I am writing this book for you.

- It will teach you how to generate more patients and revenue from your marketing.
- It will show you how you can become an expert with a celebrity aura without needing a massive PR budget or the benefit of decades in the practice.
- It will reveal how best to capitalise on your status, and how to develop it as you develop your practice.

There are seven secrets I'm about to let you in on. But for starters here's an eighth: it's actually not all that that hard.

It's time to stop flogging that dead horse.

Forget about those short cuts and start taking some smart cuts to guaranteed success.

Let's get going!

Secret #1:
How to Surpass the Established Players and Overcome the Cowboys

"The secret of business is to know something that nobody else knows."

Aristotle Onassis

There are two key threats to your practice and I'm going to show you how to overcome both of them. I've already touched on them in the Introduction: they are your competitors.

At one end of the scale are the established players and at the other end are the cowboys.

You can kick them both into touch.

The Established Specialist Surgeons

*"It's not the size of the dog in the fight.
It's the size of the fight in the dog."*

Mark Twain

Size matters, as any breast augmentation specialist will tell you. Here's how it matters to you.

When I ask the surgeons who I work with about their main competition for their favourite procedure the answer is predictable.

Sadly predictable.

Without hesitation they reel off one or two surgeons who appear to have their city's market sewn up.

Not only do these big practices carry out the majority of cases, they also charge far more than the average surgeon does for the same procedure.

It's galling isn't it? How can it be that those who charge the highest fees also have the longest waiting lists?

The response of most surgeons to this situation is one of steely resignation. They often comment glumly:

"That's just the way it is.

Dr. Ace has been around for so many years and he has all the referring doctors batting for him.

He is also the first person the press go to when they need a comment or an opinion.

It's no wonder he has all the patients: he has the reputation."

I want to tell them that it doesn't have to be this way but, before I even have a chance to speak, their fatalistic response continues:

"It's OK though.

The cosmetic surgery industry is growing fast and there are plenty of scraps still to be had.

I can make a decent living by gaining a good market share from the remainder of the patients that Dr. Ace can no longer fit in."

If you find yourself making comments like this, or just gazing enviously at other practices, then I have two things to say to you.

1. Most plastic surgeons I have met are extremely competitive, but, for some reason, they seem to throw the towel in when you mention trying to challenge the celebrity surgeons.

   The truth is, however, that you have worked too hard, and spent too many years training, to settle for second place. You should be aiming to be recognised as the best for your procedure of choice and, therefore, gaining the majority of this market share.

2. Next let's consider Dr. Ace.

   In all likelihood he has probably grown a tad lazy, like anyone who has been enjoying the spoils of victory for an extended period of time.

   I can help you pull the rug from under his feet by implementing a marketing formula that is so powerful he won't even know what has hit him.

But before we start rearranging the furniture to our liking we need to consider another challenge you are going to have to overcome: the cowboys.

The Cowboys

"Nowadays people know the price of everything, but the value of nothing."

Oscar Wilde

In your industry, more than others, there is a sizeable grey area that sits between what is legal and what is ethical.

I'm sure you don't need me to tell you that trying to compete in this grey area is a recipe for disaster, and the quickest way to engage in a race to the bottom.

We have all seen this phenomenon before: I recently witnessed it first-hand in Sydney.

For years the breast augmentation surgeons there had been living the good life. A combination of twenty years of uninterrupted Australian economic growth and ongoing demand had led to premium prices and plentiful patients.

A boob job in Sydney, according to my breast surgeon clients, used to cost up to 20% more than the same procedure in some of the most famous and well-respected cosmetic clinics in Miami, Brazil and London.

But all good things come to an end.

In early 2012, a number of new clinics opened and suddenly the prices started to tumble.

Alarmingly fast.

In no time at all they had dropped by almost 50%. It was like a whirlpool and many good practices got sucked into its inexorable downward spiral.

Here was what led to the collapse.

Many of these new clinics were operating in the grey area. They were able to cut corners by using inferior implants, by not using specialist anaesthetists and by operating in below-par facilities.

Scary, right?

Naively, a number of well-regarded plastic surgeons followed suit in a desperate effort to try and compete on price, albeit with the same high overheads they were used to paying.

I spoke to a few surgeons who actually resorted to using the 'bait and switch' tactic. This is where the doctors slashed their price simply to get patients in the door. The idea was to then upsell them to a more complex procedure, or to blindly hope that they would turn into a repeat customer.

Desperate, right?

Into this potent mix for disaster were added a large number of 'injectable' clinics. These clinics were run by general doctors who had only completed a short training course in fillers and Botox injections.

Cutting corners, dubious injection clinics and the 'bait and switch' technique are highly unethical ways to do business. In Sydney, as elsewhere, it is unfortunate that these methods proved to be highly effective ways to steer patients away from more legitimate surgeries.

These cowboys are still threatening to suck your patients away from you. Yes, they may one day end up being shut down, but it will be a bitter pill to swallow if you have closed before them because they have obliterated your cash flow.

The kind of panic response we saw in Sydney was little more than a knee-jerk reaction when what was called for was a fool-proof strategy.

You simply can't sling mud against the wall to see what sticks without dirtying your hands. This approach to marketing and advertising, when you are competing with the bottom dwellers, is a total waste of time and money.

And it just isn't effective.

The bottom end of your market offers low prices and high competition. If you do not have a plan to overcome it, as opposed to running into it head on, your clinic is in danger of either disappearing or simply becoming indistinguishable from those around it.

If you do choose to join the fray your leads will be hard to win and even harder to turn into profit. At the bottom of the barrel there is only bad credit, slim margins and 'no money down' type finance deals.

If any of the above rings true then there is no doubt that you need to implement an effective marketing strategy which can help grow your practice through trust whilst simultaneously overcoming the threat of your bottom dwelling competitors.

It can be done. You just need a plan.

A fool-proof plan.

Your A.C.E. Factor

"There is no advertisement as powerful as a positive reputation traveling fast."

Brian Koslow

Patients don't invest in high-priced procedures from Dr. Nobody. As we have seen they go to Dr. Ace.

In order for someone to pay you market-leading rates you are going to have to become a 'somebody'. But how can you do this without waiting twenty years to become established?

Life is far too short for that, so let me introduce you to the A.C.E factor.

- **A**uthority
- **C**elebrity
- **E**xpertise

One of the greatest direct marketers of our time, Dan Kennedy, coined this phrase and he has been using the theory behind it to make millions for his clients for more than thirty years.

Here's what he says about it:

"If you aren't establishing yourself as a celebrity, at least to your clientele and target market, you're asleep at the wheel.

You are ignoring what is fuelling the entire economy around you and neglecting the development of a measurably valuable asset.

The question is:

Do you have a plan you are following step-by-step to make yourself a (bigger) celebrity?

If not, why not?

If not now, when?"[i]

What are the A.C.E factor's effects?

During the height of Paris Hilton's celebrity she appeared on thirteen of the thirty covers in a magazine section. She was being paid $300,000 to appear for an hour at parties and night clubs. She became the face of several products for which she netted untold sums in licensing deals. She is, perhaps, the ultimate example of cashing in on being famous for nothing more than being famous.

The good news is that you do not need to be Paris Hilton to manufacture celebrity out of thin air.

That's a relief!

You probably have already written journals or papers to further your professional education or gain you promotions or status. You have also trained for many years perfecting your craft.

You are a highly trained medical professional.

That's more than a start!

You already have the expertise and the authority: all that's missing is the celebrity.

So let's establish it.

When you have the A.C.E factor, you will be so far ahead of the pack that it's unlikely anyone will ever be able to get near you.

When you're a hot commodity you can keep your prices at a level which works for you, and still have patients seeking you out.

You will make better margins on your procedures, so you can afford to work less and spend more time with your family.

So, what do you actually need to do to develop your A.C.E factor?

The answer is so simple you may not believe it at first, but bear with me because I know it works.

And I can show you exactly how.

But first you are going to need to transform yourself into a published author.

You didn't expect that did you?

The Benefits of Becoming a Published Author

"There is no friend as loyal as a book."

Ernest Hemingway

Why on earth should you write a book?

I understand this idea may appear slightly off the wall. I am going to show you why it works, how you can do it and how you can use it to transform your marketing and the success of your practice.

Your initial incredulity is understandable, however.

First let me assure that this is not a vanity publishing exercise that results in a book that no-one will read. Many people will read your book and many more will become your patients directly as a result.

This is not a tangent or a side line either. It is the very heart of what will help you compete with the celebrity surgeons and separate yourself once and for all from the cowboys.

The seven marketing secrets that I'm about to reveal to you are all built around the concept of transforming you into a published author and leveraging the benefits this gives you to set yourself apart.

Your book will be the stone thrown into the pond whose ripples will spread and grow larger.

If you can't see it yet you are going to have to bear with me, because you don't want to miss out on this.

Trust me.

Let me just try and help you visualise how it works.

What you hold in your hands is your proof. You received this book didn't you? You are reading it right now, aren't you?

Well, I use this book to reach my audience of cosmetic surgeons like yourself. I engage them with it and many will appreciate my advice: they will reach out to me and ask for my help. I don't even really need to even ask them to contact me. They just do because they know that I understand their market and I have shown them how to crack it.

In essence I am asking you to do exactly what I do. And I wouldn't do it if it didn't work.

In this book I am giving you really useful information. I hope this will earn your respect and gain your trust. In doing so it's only natural that you will turn to me when you need advice. If you don't but I have gained your respect I am also happy. You will tell others about me. And so it goes on.

This book is not just about a marketing strategy: it is an actual example of how this strategy works.

Let me now explain further the five key benefits of writing a book to you.

1. Trust and credibility

You are not aiming to get rich from the sales of your book, although that would be nice. As a matter of fact I am actually going to advise you to give copies of your book out for free. (Oh dear, have I just lost what little faith I had instilled in you?)

What you are going to get rich from is the trust and credibility that will result from being an author of a well-written, extremely helpful book.

When someone reads your book, and they learn exactly how you can help them, you will instantly gain the A.C.E factor.

An author is an authority.

A cosmetic surgeon who is an author is also unique. Check out Amazon for other books about cosmetic surgery that are aimed at consumers rather than practitioners. You will find only a handful: you are about to join these elite few.

2. Recognition

As an author you will find the press suddenly start calling on you. Great news!

Your peers will spontaneously invite you to speak at conferences and conventions. Great reputation enhancement!

What's more referring doctors will begin to take you seriously. Great numbers of pre-qualified prospects!

Books can open doors (and not just as doorstops).

3. Patient generation

This is where it really counts.

You are not writing a book to stroke your ego but to skyrocket your patient numbers.

Think for a second about your website.

- How many visitors does it get each month?
- And how many of these make an enquiry?
- How many of these enquiries become consultations?
- And how many of these actually undergo treatment?

There are just so many ways the journey from interest to patient can breakdown, and a book published by yourself can fix them. Not in every case, of course, but in sufficient numbers to make a real difference to your business.

Let's remember that a key effect of producing a book is a healthy injection of trust and credibility into your proposition. It could be the element that wipes away any lingering doubts.

Now let's imagine that you're advising a patient about the merits of breast augmentation. They are with you, but not 100% with you.

As they leave you offer them a complimentary copy of your book, commenting that many others have said it helped them think the whole thing through.

You schedule a call for next week, and you know you have played your most powerful card in the deck. You have won their trust, positioned yourself as an authority and gained their good will.

That's a powerful mix indeed.

In addition you have given them a book that will answer all their questions and soothe any lasting concerns.

That's a winning formula.

4. Prospecting with Amazon

Your book, however, is more than a conversion tool. It is also a prospecting tool, and there is plenty of gold up in them there hills.

Later on I'm going to show you just how powerful your book can be when used to generate prospects online. Right now I want to show you how your book will allow you to harness the online visibility and trust of Amazon and use it to your advantage.

When people are unsure about something they look for help. They may turn to a friend, a colleague or a specialist. They are equally likely these days to look online. One thing that people trust as a source of information is the written word. And where do you look for books online? You make a search on Amazon.

Here's the thing about Amazon. Once again, I'm not going to tell you that you are about to become a bestselling author: this is not part of our game plan. I am going to tell you, however, that people often search for information on Amazon: whether or not they buy the books they find is irrelevant to us. The fact that your book will be there makes a profound difference to your credibility.

And credibility brings enquiries.

5. Protecting your reputation

There are obvious ways that a book helps to build your reputation. There are less obvious ways that it can protect it.

I'm sure you know how easy it is to receive the odd bad review online. You are also probably painfully aware of how this one bad apple can literally spoil the rest of the reviews in your cart.

I'm going to show you just how you can build your reputation online later. For now I'd like you to consider how just having a book can protect it.

People search for reviews by typing your name into a search engine: up pops your website, your social media profiles and usually some review sites.

Now let's assume they do the same search after you have published your book. What dominates the first page of the search results now will be your website, your social media profiles, your Amazon listing and press reviews of your book. The review sites will probably be pushed onto the second page.

First impressions count. Before your prospect even reaches the occasional bad review they will know you are a widely respected author, an expert in your field and an authority figure.

And that will help take the sting out of any negative reviews that may lurk out there.

How to Publish Your Book

"A book is a gift you can open again and again."

Garrison Keillor

Hopefully I have shown you that this is not a madcap scheme.

It is a genuine, highly effective strategy that will set you apart and win you patients.

So, let's get down to the nitty-gritty.

You may wonder how you are expected to find the time to write a book in the first place. Well, I'm going to outline here how you can become an author in as little as five hours of your time.

That's right five hours.

All you need is a little help from your practice manager or secretary, and a few very special online tools.

We need to be absolutely clear on one thing. Your book is definitely not going to be all about you. When most people write books they are writing about themselves.

- Me, Me, Me.
- What I can do for you.
- Here is what I do.
- Here is how I do it.
- This is the best thing ever.

Your book will be different.

It will be written from your typical prospect's point of view. It will address and answer their questions.

- What's in it for them?
- What do they get out of the book?
- What can they do?
- How can they do it?
- What's best for them?

By answering their questions your book will be the best thing ever without ever needing to proclaim itself as such.

Now let's get this book written.

Writing a book in less than five hours of your time is easier than you might think. And you can do it.

Here's how.

Step #1: Choose your procedure

Your book should focus on just one procedure. This will help it find its market and help you establish your reputation.

Step #2: Profile your patient

- Who is your ideal or typical patient?
- Are they male or female?
- How old are they?
- Where do they live?
- Do they have children?
- Is there an income level demographic?
- Are they conservative or liberal?
- What do they read, watch or enjoy doing?

- What are their hope, fears, dreams and pain?
- Why do they want surgery?

Take your time on this and write it all down, because you will be using this information later.

Step #3: Chart the territory

Write down around twenty statements that solve common problems for your profile patient or things that they may ask as questions about the particular procedure you are focussing on.

This should be really easy for you because you most likely answer these sorts of questions every single day.

Step #4: Come up with the big idea

Once you have these questions written down have a slow read through them.

You are looking for common themes that unite these issues and you are going to use this to come up with the big idea that will form the focus of your book.

What exactly will your book do?

Does it offer 'The truth about Botox'? Does it provide 'The ultimate guide to breast augmentation'?

Once you have your big idea you are ready to start structuring and writing your book.

Step #5: Plot your book

Grab ten index cards.

On each of them write down one question, objection or challenge that relates to your big idea. These are most likely to be your ten best questions or statements that you identified in Step #2 above.

Now write three prompt words on the back of each card: these are to remind you how to answer the question posed on the front.

Read through what you have and pick your favourite seven out of the ten. You now have your seven chapters that will form the basis of what you are going to write. Order them as logically as possible from one through to seven and you have plotted out the structure of your book.

Step #6: Start fleshing out the detail

We're not finished with those index cards yet!

Take four more cards for each of your seven chapters. On each card write down a 'subheading'. These are going to be the sections that make up each chapter.

Here's an example to make it crystal clear what you are to do for this step.

- Chapter: 'How do I choose a breast surgeon?'
- Subheading #1: 'Are they registered with the relevant plastic surgeon societies?'
- Subheading #2: 'Do they operate in accredited facilities?'

- Subheading #3: 'What types of breast implants do they use?'
- Subheading #4: 'Do they work as a specialist at major teaching hospitals?'

Do this for all seven questions relying on your knowledge of the sorts of questions you are asked every day.

Step #7: Introduce yourself

And we're off! It's time to start writing, but don't worry you only need fill a couple of pages.

The first page will be the introduction to your book. It only literally needs to be about a page long.

Here's what you need to write.

- Start by introducing yourself and what your qualifications are.
  - o What are your accolades?
  - o What makes you an expert?
- Then tell your story.
  - o Why did you get into cosmetic surgery?
  - o Why did you decide to specialise in this particular procedure? Why are you different to your competitors?
- Now you need to let your reader know a couple of things.
  - o Who this book is for?
  - o What problems it will solve?
- Finally you simply need to say, 'Let's get started'.

Step #8: Record yourself

This is where the real magic happens.

You are now going to record yourself answering the questions you have written down on the index cards.

The best way to do this is to use the rather amazing SpeakWrite app (speakwrite.com). It's a free service, so why not download it now and have a play.

As you record yourself don't worry about mistakes, hesitations or 'umms' and 'ahhs'. Just speak freely into your phone and answer the questions in as much detail as you can.

Once you have done this you can breathe a sigh of relief: you are almost there.

Step #9: Wrap things up

All that is left is to write an ending for your book. Again, this need only be one page and here is the tried and tested formula you can follow.

- Recap what was covered in each of your chapters.
- Tell the reader they can now feel confident to take action using the tips you have given them.
- And, finally, include a call to action:
  'If you want to move forward with a consultation on XYZ go to my website example.com, or pick up the phone and dial...'

The rest of the work on your book need not involve you.

Easy wasn't it?

Step #10: Get it in writing

You can pay a transcribing service to turn the audio recordings you have made into text. This is likely to cost no more than $1USD per minute, and, if you use SpeakWrite's excellent transcription service to turn your audio into text, it takes just three hours.

Step #11: Sit back and let someone else finish your work

Once you receive the transcript in Word format you can find yourself an editor who will tidy it all up for you.

Services such as Odesk (www.odesk.com) or Elance (www.elance.com) can provide a professional editor for around $100-$200USD. The editor will take the complete text file, your introduction and ending and they will put it all together so that it reads well and is in a logical order.

And there you have it.

A well-written book, crammed with useful information, just waiting to be published. It should come in at about 75-100 pages so this is no lightweight tome but a heavyweight contender.

Stop the clock!

It has taken you personally no more than five hours to do this. So what are we waiting for?

Let's get this book published.

Getting the Cover Designed

"Cover art serves one purpose and one purpose only: to get potential customers interested. In the internet age this means the thumbnail image needs to be interesting enough to click on. That's what covers are for."

Larry Correia

You could be spending a small fortune designing artwork and amazing graphics for your book. But, with a little help from the web, there is no real need for this.

What I always recommend to my clients is to search out a life-saving website called Fiverr (www.fiverr.com). If you haven't visited this site before, you'll be amazed at what you can get done there for $5USD. It offers you an instant portal to a whole other world in which people will do a vast amount of work for a 'fiver'. And they do it well.

So you can get your book cover designed here with no fuss whatsoever. There are only a couple of things to bear in mind.

The first is to make sure you search for 'book cover designs' rather than '3D eBooks'. You should also make it absolutely clear to the person who will design your cover that you want this for a printed book.

When you place your order the service provider will give you clear instructions about all they need from you. This is where you need to make certain that they understand your requirements. Your most important requirement is simple: you want the title and strapline to stand-out on the cover. These are your most important element, not the graphics, background pattern or anything else.

Let me explain this a bit further because it is absolutely crucial. You are going to be taking photos of you holding your book for use on your website, which means that the cover will be small and hard to read, so the title needs to be prominent. Your book cover will also appear as a thumbnail image on Amazon, in press coverage and elsewhere. You need a bold title.

You will get the design returned within a day, and now it's time to let the print presses roll and start putting your book to work.

You might need to spend a bit more time to get a high-quality file made from the file you receive from the designer. This is known as a 'PSD' file and is the sort of file that your printer will need.

Your printed book is just one step away from being in your hands and you are just moments away from starting to gain the A.C.E factor and secure your surgery's entry into the elite league.

Getting Your Book Printed

"The printing press is the greatest weapon in the armoury of the modern commander."

T. E. Lawrence

CreateSpace (www.createspace.com) is owned by Amazon and it is definitely the best place to get your book published. It's cheap, it offers great quality printing and its links with Amazon offer all kinds of bonus benefits you simply can't afford to miss out on.

You are looking at approximately $2USD for each black and white paperback book you print, and you can order as few as ten copies at a time.

In addition you can get your book set up to be read on a Kindle at the same time as it is printed. CreateSpace also allows you to set your book up to be sold on Amazon as well. Its quick to do and it couldn't be easier.

If you've followed the process that has been outlined then you will already have all the pieces of the puzzle in place. All you need to do now is create an account and login: CreateSpace will walk you through the rest of the process step-by-step.

A piece of cake really!

So what's next?

- You have positioned yourself as an expert in your field. You are a published author and very few, if any, of your competitors can claim to be this.
  (Share your book with as many prospects as you can!)

- You will soon become a first choice amongst doctors who want to refer their patients to the best plastic surgeon offering your procedure.
  (Share your book with as many doctors as you can!)

- You will also be the go-to surgeon for local and national television news shows, radio shows, newspapers and magazines looking for an expert opinion.
  (Share your book with as many journalists as you can!)

- You can have copies of your book in your waiting rooms, and give it away as consultations close.
  (Just think what that will do to your consultation to surgery conversion percentage?)

- You can give your book away as a marketing tactic to ensure you capture a prospective patient's name and email address.
  (I will show you exactly how to do this later.)

- You can proudly show a photo of you and your book on your website.
  (Not just for an ego-boost but to greatly improve your Google AdWords campaign conversions and profitability. Remember that your book gives you the A.C.E factor.)

- Plus much, much more.
  (Which I'll outline for you as we reach the other six of my seven secrets of patient generation.)

All of a sudden this book idea begins to make a lot more sense doesn't it?

So many times I have seen the incredulous faces on clients when the idea is first introduced. For those brave enough to give it a go I have seen the results return for every single one.

There is only space here to offer you a brief outline of the process, but it makes a beautiful sketch nonetheless. All that it needs is for you to paint your own canvas from it.

Here's the real takeaway. This is all in your grasp. Creating a fantastic book that your patients want to read is not as hard or as time consuming as it sounds.

But it will deliver results.

Gaining yourself the A.C.E factor just needs a decision from you to not follow the herd and to do something different. Authority, expertise and celebrity status are yours for the taking.

And you will leave those cowboys eating your dust.

Getting Your Book in the Hands of Your Prospects

"Build it and they will come."

Kevin Costner,
in the film 'Field of Dreams'

Have you ever heard this phrase used? It's visionary, it's romantic, it's poetic... and it's completely untrue.

'Build it and they will come' is from one of my favourite films of all time. 'Field of Dreams' starred Kevin Costner and Ray Liotta: I just can't believe it was made in 1989! How time has flown.

Sadly, for many, not a lot has changed. There are still far too many surgeons believing that you can simply build it and they will come. As if a cosmetic surgery practice somehow just markets itself!

- Spend a fortune on a website and patients will find me.
- Spend a fortune on consulting rooms and patients will fill them.
- Spend a fortune hiring the best practice manager and things will just miraculously fall into place.

These are all prime examples of ways to fail.

The same is going to be true when it comes to promoting your book. Having a book is one thing: using it effectively is another.

You are going to need to work hard at getting your new paperback book into the hands of your prospective patients.

Here are some tips to make it easier for you and highly effective for your practice.

Using Magazines and Local Newspapers

Remember when I asked you to profile your ideal customer so you understood who you were writing your book for? I asked you to consider what magazines they flicked through and what newspapers they read.

There was a reason for that. You can use a special one page printed piece detailing your free book giveaway. In the trade it's known as a free standing insert and it offers a powerful way to market yourself. Here's the best bit: hardly anyone in your industry is taking advantage of it.

The free standing insert does what is says on the tin: it sits within the paper and falls out when someone gives it a jiggle.

This 8.5 x 11 inch piece of paper can be used in several different ways.

- It can be used in your local newspaper.
- It could be used as a flyer that you pay someone to deliver around town.
- You could use it as the basis of a full page ad in a magazine.
- You could put it in an envelope and mail it.

Use Postcards Because You Wish They Were Here

Postcards are a great way to drive leads. You can use them to send people to the landing page on your website that gives the book away in exchange for a name, email and full postal address.

And now you have their details to keep up a conservation and create a consultation.

You can use your in-house database to send out a postcard with details of your new book and an invitation to get it for free. You'll be amazed at how it offers the most effective way to spark up a meaningful conversation.

Use Facebook Advertising

I have devoted a whole chapter to Facebook advertising later in this book for the simple reason that it is the fastest way to get your message to anyone you desire. And it costs next to nothing.

Your book is central to this game-changing plan.

Use Forum Advertising Opportunities

In both the UK and Australia there are many online forums that act as a place for patients to share their stories and recommend surgeons. It's true that they are also spaces to criticise surgeons so, as a side-note, someone in your team should be trawling these monthly to make sure there isn't a shockingly bad review by a disgruntled patient.

The great news is that the people who hang out on these forums are almost guaranteed to be ready to book their consultation. They are making their final decisions at the very end of their customer journey.

This is why these forums are *the* places to get your brand in front of the best type of prospects.

Most forums carry advertising. They offer some very competitive rates for banner advertising within these forums – all you have to do is reach out and negotiate a price.

Get a banner designed (remembering that you can do these sorts of things quickly and cost-effectively at <u>fiverr.com</u>). Use your banner to advertise your free book, and then make the banner link to the landing page on your website where you offer your book.

The webmaster from the forum will look after the rest. That is after they have taken payment, of course!

Hire an Email Database

I don't care what procedure you are promoting: someone out there will have an email database available for rent. You should be using it to let people know about your free book.

When I say rent I mean that you will have to pay them £500 (or around $1000 AUD) to send an email to their database of, say, 2000 qualified contacts.

Just think: if 800 people open up your email, and 10% of these raise their hand you can bet it will be money well spent.

If you are struggling to find a list just go back to your ideal prospect you created for your book.

- Where do they spend time online?
- What local gyms do they visit?
- Which are the main cosmetic clinics they buy their facial products from?

There are plenty of options waiting for you: if you can start to really get to know and understand your patients.

You needn't worry that by using email lists you are about to become a spammer. This is, of course, one of the last things that you want to do. Thanks to your book you have set yourself apart once and for all from the cowboys who send 'spammy' mails to try and gain new patients. You are offering a free, quality educational book, not a cut-price procedure. Those interested will respond because they appreciate the chance to learn more, and you will know that those who do respond are seriously considering surgery.

Six Other Secrets That Will Unleash Your Patient Generation Potential

"Most of us have experienced wow moments. We just haven't taken time to think deeply about them."

Michael Hyatt

Your book is not a piece of vanity publishing. It is going to be central to the marketing and success of your practice. It is a business decision but one you are going to really enjoy taking. I know you are going to love 'writing' the book, seeing it in print and seeing the difference it makes to your status, consultations and patient numbers.

Your book is the keystone that you will build your bridges around. In the next few chapters I'm going to open things out a little and reveal some more secrets that will help you reach your prospects, nurture them and convert them into patients.

At the centre of everything you are about to do will be your book, the A.C.E factor and the competitive advantage you gain by choosing to be bold and original in your marketing.

You are not here to play the game only. You are here to win the game: you will do this by changing the rules. Let's look at how you can shake things up so well that you ensure all the pieces land to your advantage.

Secret #2:
How to Nurture Your Existing Database and Grow Your Lists

"If you build it... you may still need Google AdWords to make them come."

Jennifer Mesenbrink

I have been helping plastic surgery clinics skyrocket their qualified lead lists for many years. It's what I do.

In 2014 alone I delivered:

- 50 million ad impressions and 350,000 clicks on Facebook's advertising platform.
- 8.5 million ad impressions and 172,000 clicks on Google AdWords.

But here's the rub.

For every 100 leads that are generated through your spend on ads there are, on average, five or less that will convert into patients.

So what happens to the other 95 you pay to acquire?

Let's not be too negative: in truth the five surgeries you have gained are great and will help you achieve a fair return on your investment. It's just that the true value of your investment probably lies in the 95 prospective patients you have gained, and not in the five patients.

Your clinic *must* nurture these prospects if your leads are going to actually lead anywhere.

Consider this: 80% of 'bookings' are made somewhere between the fifth and the twelfth contact.

Only very few are made on the first.

By nurturing and following up on leads you have the opportunity to build trust with prospects, make them feel comfortable with you and gain a booking from what would otherwise appear as wasted ad spend.

But to do this you must have a plan. If you think having your secretary make a phone call when they get the lead, and then scheduling a follow up call in a few weeks is good enough, you are in trouble.

Yet, amazingly, this is all most cosmetic surgery practices actually do. The industry seems to be miles behind others, and not many of your competitors are taking lead nurturing seriously at all.

This is your chance to place yourself ahead of the pack.

Let's look at what you need to do to nurture your prospects and turn them into patients.

The first thing is to make contact in many different ways. One form of media is not enough because people process and respond to types of communication differently. Some prefer visual communication, some respond better to hearing and some are more apt to consider the printed word. This means that if you use just email, you are missing out on a big opportunity.

A relatively small amount of work will make a huge difference to the number of leads that you see becoming patients.

Here are a few ways you can start communicating effectively and making your ad spend continue to work for you long after that click became a lead.

Send Everyone on Your List a Copy of Your Book

"The best marketing doesn't feel like marketing."

Tom Fishburne

By now it should be clear: you need to develop your celebrity status by becoming a published author. Once this is done, get the book printed and send a free signed copy in the post to everyone on your existing patient database.

You have now lit the touch paper. Sit back and enjoy the fireworks.

Set Up an Email Autoresponder

"Good marketing makes the company look smart.
Great marketing makes the customer feel smart."

Joe Chernov

Setting up an email autoresponder saves you time and makes you money. It ensures that you are sending out your most effective emails to your list every single time and it helps educate your prospects whilst leading them step-by-step to your consulting room.

Autoresponders keep on working so you don't have to. They deliver you a constant supply of new enquiries from your leads without so much as the need to hit 'send'.

You have heard of Mailchimp or AWeber, right? If not, then look them up: they are about to transform your email communication's conversion potential.

All you need to do to achieve this is the following.

1. Re-use some of the educational content from your book or from your previous blog posts.
2. Load them up into an autoresponder.
3. Pre-program them to go out to your database every week or so for as long as you want.
4. If you want to get really smart you could even set up your favourite mails to automatically go out to any new leads that are added to your database so that everyone receives your most effective communications first.

That's it. Enjoy the results.

Strong Words, Softly Spoken: the Power of Audio

"The voice of the intellect is a soft one, but it must not rest until it has gained a hearing."

Sigmund Freud

By using the methods mentioned earlier to record yourself narrating your book you will have already created a CD that your prospects can listen to in their cars on their way to work.

All it needs is a little editing and you have another powerful marketing tool waiting to be used.

Get the CD sent, along with a quick note, in the post to your database, and they will love your for it. Not everyone will take the time to read a book but we can all grab a few moments here and there to listen to one.

Get your audiobook out there and let the patients start coming in.

How to Write the Perfect Newsletter

"Content builds relationships. Relationships are built on trust. Trust drives revenue."

Andrew Davis

This tip is so important it should be implemented right away within your practice. If you do not send out a follow up newsletter already you are missing out on a huge opportunity.

Why is it so important?

Most prospects are not ready to go ahead with surgery when they first contact you. That book in the mail, that click on an AdWords campaign or that exploratory phone call are very much first steps, and there may be a long way to travel alongside them before they become a patient.

You need to stay in front of your prospects for as long as possible, and they live a busy life too! It may seem hard to believe but you are very soon going to be far from the front of their minds.

Breast reduction and abdominoplasty patients, for example, are notorious for their painstaking research and the length of time it takes them to decide on surgery. They are only going to go ahead with surgery when they are 100% ready, and you need to stay with them all the way if they are going to choose to become your patient.

Regular, quality communication is a must. It builds trust, offers ongoing opportunities to take the next step and keeps you front of mind. Be consistent by sending out a newsletter to the people in your database every single month.

Make sure you send it to them via email as well as in the post. Remember that each contact may respond more positively to different means of communication. As a minimum you need to plan for a follow up campaign that lasts a year, but there is a good argument for continuing to maintain contact beyond this.

This is another marketing essential that, for some reason, others in your industry are not doing. By sending out a monthly newsletter you will once more be giving your practice a huge advantage.

It is highly unlikely that there is just one prospect on your database that has not also been in contact with another practice. It is also highly likely that many of these other practices are not keeping in contact in a consistent, structured way. It's their loss and you can make it your gain.

By keeping in contact, and keeping yourself front of mind, when your prospect is ready to go ahead it's highly probable you will be the only practice that has remained in regular contact. Who do you think they will choose?

Ideas for Content to Include in Your Newsletter

The importance of a monthly newsletter is beyond doubt, but it somewhat begs the question of what you will find to put in it. Exactly what information should your practice include in its monthly missives?

It's true that on the face of it generating ideas for newsletters can seem daunting. In the same way the thought of writing a book seemed like being asked to plan an ascent up Everest. I'm going to show you how newsletters need not take up much time but will pay you back several times over for the investment you make.

Here are some simple ways you can find ideas for things to write about and some sure-fire tips on making sure they will be interesting, engaging, memorable and, ultimately, convincing for your prospective patients.

1. 'Letter from the surgeon'
   This is a great way to humanise your clinic and make your prospects develop connections with you.

2. 'Patient story'
   A patient telling their story is extremely powerful and can be used as a 'testimonial' for your practice.

3. 'Employee spotlight'
   Like the 'letter from the surgeon' having a newsletter which profiles your injecting nurses or practice manager can humanise your clinic.

4. Company news
   Have you recently helped a charity? Appeared on TV? Extended your practice? Spoke at an event? Reached a milestone? Make these stories the themes for some of your monthly newsletters.

5. Editorials

   These thought-pieces will reflect the surgeon's views on a particular subject. For example, you may comment on the latest trends behind the gimmick 'stem cell facelifts'. It helps position you as an expert and informs your prospects about the issue in question and your status as a reliable source of information.

6. Blog excerpts

   If you publish awesome blog content, extend its life by sharing excerpts from it in your newsletter. This could be as a one-off article or a regular feature that profiles the top five blog posts of the month. If they work online they are sure to engage in a newsletter!

7. Special offers

   If you have special offers then a newsletter is a really great place to talk about them. You can even time their announcement with the newsletter so that your database is given priority treatment.

8. Q&A

   If one person asks a question, there is no doubt that others will be thinking about the same thing. Take your most frequently asked questions and answer them within your newsletter. Again you can do this as a one-off article or as a regular feature.

9. New service announcements
    Have you recently employed a new injecting nurse? Or are you about to introduce Botox into your list of services? Write about the launch and make your prospects feel special about being the first to know about the new procedure.

10. Event calendar
    Many surgeons appear at conferences or expos which are planned months in advance. Tell your database about these dates. It simply builds up your A.C.E factor further.

11. Case studies or white papers
    These are more in-depth looks at how your procedures have helped your patients and usually include bits of information taken from the latest research. They help once again to establish you as someone with their finger on the pulse.

12. Before and after photos
    It doesn't all have to be words, words, words. If you have recently snapped any great before and afters be sure to add them to your newsletter.

How to Structure Your Newsletter

By now you should be brimming with ideas for content so the benefits of a newsletter are firmly within your grasp, but how are you going to design it?

There's no need to reinvent the wheel: I have used a design template that looks great and works like a dream and you can feel free to use it.

Rather than go into detail about how to design the perfect two-page newsletter, I have simply gone ahead and provided the template design that I use so that you can use for your practice.

Simply download it and there can be no more excuses! All I ask is that send you me a quick email so I know just how well it's working for you.

You can download this design here goo.gl/0DMDJd

And email me at dan@flexxdigital.com in a few months' time.

An Easy Way to Re-ignite a Dead Database

"When it is obvious that the goals cannot be reached, don't adjust the goals, adjust the action steps."

Confucius

There will always be some prospects in your database that just don't seem to be responding anymore. Here's a simple but effective 'reactivation' email that I learnt from a famous marketer named Dean Jackson.

Dean's original email contained just nine words and was sent to real estate leads.

It read:

"Are you still looking for a house in Georgetown?"

That's it. Nothing more. It's short and to the point yet it re-engages your dormant prospects like a dream.

I use variations of it all the time for dormant leads. You know, those people who have already been introduced to a clinic, made an initial connection, but then have not shown the slightest bit of interest.

How well does it work? Well, I've found open rates on these emails are 15-200% higher than what should be typically expected for the list. Bear in mind that it is sent to a seemingly 'dead' section of the database too.

Here's the template I use (and it's so simple there's no need to download it):

Subject

(name of prospect)

Nine-word body

('Are you still interested in our face lift package?' or 'Are you still interested in a breast augmentation consultation?')

No more, no less. You don't even need to include your name or a salutation at the end. That's how well it works.

Give it a go: you will be surprised by the response you receive. And with significantly more active prospects now on your list you will also be pleasantly surprised by the patients that result.

Survey Your Prospects

"To think creatively, we must be able to look afresh at what we normally take for granted."

George Kneller

Surveys are another trick of the trade that I regularly use for all my surgeons, and it works like gangbusters. What's more I place my survey on pages on their websites that are usually no more than a waste of space.

Surveys can convert functional web pages into prime online real estate. They can also convert simple enquiries into highly qualified prospects.

You may wonder just how a survey can help you to achieve this. Let's take a second and think about it.

- Completing a survey bonds your prospect further to your business.
- It provides you with stacks of useful information about them. It tells you exactly what queries they have and what barriers may need to be overcome. It even gives you extra ways to get in contact such as a phone number or mailing address.
- Finally, it gives you the perfect reason to get back in contact with them.

Here's an example of a survey that I placed the 'thank-you page' for a plastic surgeon client in Sydney:

THANK YOU

Thanks for contacting us!

We will be in touch within one business working day. If you need to get in touch urgently please call us on ████████████

In the meantime, we would love to know more about you – please complete the following survey so we can improve our patient satisfaction.

Let us learn more about you.

The below survey will take 2 minutes of your time. it will help us understand more about you before we get in touch.

*Required

Image deleted for client confidentiality.

Name *

What Cosmetic procedure are you looking for? *
ie Neck Lift, Tummy Tuck, Eyelid Surgery, Rhinoplasty etc etc

Have you had any cosmetic procedures before? If so, can you please list below.

Do you have a time frame for your procedure?

In this survey the patient actually provides details about their time frame for potential surgery, which is invaluable information for understanding how best to market your services.

Hang on a minute, though.

This survey was placed on a 'thank-you page'? What on earth is a survey doing on a 'thank-you page'?

What it is doing is transforming a dead page into a powerful marketing tool.

Let me explain exactly how this simple but highly effective little 'trick' works.

1. The prospect finds your website and enquiry form via the usual marketing channels (AdWords, Facebook, SEO etc.).
2. They fill in the enquiry form and are then redirected to a 'thank-you page'.
3. The 'thank-you page' is pre-populated with your survey.

A 'thank-you page' usually says 'thanks for getting in touch, we will call you within one business working day', or some similar fluff that is equally boring and a complete waste of both your, and your prospect's, time. When faced with such a page your prospect has only one option: to close their internet browser and continue on their merry way.

What a waste!

There could not be a better opportunity to find out more about them than right now. After all they have just taken the time to complete an enquiry form. They are interested in your service and they are in the right frame of mind to tell you about themselves.

That's why you need a survey form waiting for them.

Does it work? It truly does: I find that on average about 60% of the people landing on the 'thank-you page' go on to provide my practices with invaluable marketing information about themselves.

That is an astounding percentage. And you can get all this from them:

- An alternate phone number.
- Their time frame.
- Details of their history.
- In fact, whatever you ask.

You can do this for your business *today* without any effort at all.

There are many tools out there that can create surveys for you, with no programming experience required and often no costs at all. Wufoo (www.wufoo.com) and Survey Monkey (www.surveymonkey.com) are two popular options, but I use Google Forms because it's highly effective, simple to use and completely free.

Here's how you can do the same.

1. Type in https://drive.google.com/ into your browser (making sure you are logged into your Google account).

2. Click the 'Create' button in the top left, then 'Form'.

3. In the form template that opens, you can add any question you like and design your form by adding headers, logos and photos.

4. Click 'Send form', grab the code and place it on your website.

Job done. It couldn't be easier.

And this little hack allows you to learn from your future customers.

A Little Bit of Hard Work

"It's hard to beat a person who never gives up."

Babe Ruth

I'm going to make you a promise.

When you implement all of these different ways to nurture your prospects you are going to experience a big spike in new patients.

If it all seems a bit daunting right now it's important that you keep your eyes on the prize. Surgeons know better than most that a little bit of hard work never hurt anyone.

The beauty is that it's actually not all that hard, and all the work you put in will soon be forgotten as soon as the results start to happen.

And they will. I know because I have seen it time after time.

Now you have established your reputation and nurtured your prospects you are going to need to make sure you protect what you have worked so hard to build.

Let's talk about how reviews can make or break your standing.

Secret #3:
Building Your Online Reputation with Independent Reviews

"Your brand name is only as good as your reputation."

Richard Branson

We all know of those surgeons who operate within the grey areas of cosmetic surgery. Paradoxically they, more than anyone, understand the importance of reviews and testimonials. To an extent, that is.

Take one quick look at their websites and you will find glowing reviews and testimonials. Take a closer look at you can identify several that are clearly spurious and many that are illegal.

The Reviewing Rules

"Reputation, reputation, reputation! Oh, I have lost my reputation! I have lost the immortal part of myself, and what remains is bestial."

William Shakespeare

In both the UK and Australian markets that I work in there are strict rules when it comes to publishing reviews on your website. I probably don't need to remind you of the details of these, but below is a quick recap.

Australia

The Australian regulations are very strict indeed: quite simply testimonials are forbidden on cosmetic surgeons' websites.

The Australian Society of Plastic Surgeons (ASPS) clearly outlines this amongst other rules.

"Currently in Australia, it is not illegal for a medical practitioner (e.g. a GP) to perform surgery. It is legal for doctors with only a Bachelor's degree, such as a Bachelor of Medicine and Bachelor of Surgery (MBBS) degree, to perform. Consumers should also beware of unethical advertising practices. Some common unacceptable advertising tactics include:

- *Misleading use of professional titles i.e. giving the impression of having qualification or training in an area that the practitioner does not have;*

- *Creating unrealistic expectations through misleading or deceptive 'before' and 'after' images;*
- *Encouraging inappropriate, indiscriminate, unnecessary or excessive use of health services e.g. 'don't delay', 'achieve the look you want today';*
- *Using testimonials or purported testimonials;*
- *Offering gifts, discounts and promotions for services, and using phrases like 'as low as' or 'lowest prices'.*[vii]

United Kingdom

The policies in the UK are a little more relaxed concerning testimonials, however documentary evidence for them is required.

The CAP (Committee of Advertising Practice) Code states that:

"3.45 Marketers must hold documentary evidence that a testimonial or endorsement used in a marketing communication is genuine, unless it is obviously fictitious, and hold contact details for the person who, or organisation that, gives it.

3.46 Testimonials must relate to the advertised product.

3.47 Claims that are likely to be interpreted as factual and appear in a testimonial must not mislead or be likely to mislead the consumer."[viii]

Reviews and Testimonials on Independent Websites

"Reputation is only a candle. You still need matches to make it worth."

Paul Coehlo

Let me ask you a few simple questions:

- Do you know what your patients are saying about you online?
- Do you have a strong five star reputation?
- Are you personally responding to negative reviews?
- Do you have a strategy to gain more five star reviews?

I don't need to tell you how thorough prospective patients can be when researching their surgeon. One of the very first things your prospects will do is visit Google and type in 'your name + reviews'. If you don't already know what they will find now is the time to see for yourself what your online reputation looks like.

The results can make or break your ability to increase the number of patients who arrive at your practice. All those advertising dollars could be going to waste if you fall at the first hurdle after an initial clickthrough.

If your prospective patients can't find you or, even worse, if all they see are negative reviews, I am afraid that usually they will move onto the next surgeon they are thinking of seeing for a consultation.

If you are lucky, they may visit a forum to ask if anyone else has had a procedure with you. Here is an actual question taken from a UK forum:

"Part of me thinks he is the expert, and so maybe I should relax a little and let him have the final say, but I haven't been able to find 'any' reviews online about him or his work. I have looked everywhere..."

If you aren't well established, or if you haven't operated on a lot of patients for the procedure in question, it is unlikely you will ever see this prospect becoming one of your patients. And they won't be the only one that fails to make it.

So, how do you build your online reputation?

My recommendation is to turn to these websites:

1. http://www.google.co.uk/business/go/index.html (UK) or www.google.com.au/mybusiness (AU)

2. www.realself.com (UK and AU)

3. www.thegoodsurgeonguide.co.uk (UK)

4. www.freeindex.co.uk (UK)

5. www.plasticsurgeryhub.com.au (AU)

6. au.doctorinspector.com (AU)

7. www.doctoralia.com.au (AU)

8. www.healthengine.com.au (AU)

Local directories like these offer the opportunity for your post-op patients to review your services honestly, and recommend you in a 'testimonial' format that is approved, and even endorsed, by the search engines. These are the websites that will appear on the first page of Google when someone types in your name.

Testimonials are so credible because they were posted voluntarily on independent websites. Everyone understands that here people can be upfront and honest about their experience with you and the service they received. This is so much more powerful than an anonymous testimonial on your own website that anyone could have posted or fabricated out of thin air. Remember your potential patients aren't stupid and they are looking for concrete proof they can trust you.

We all know that genuine online testimonials are of great value: they are the digital equivalent of word of mouth referrals.

But how can you secure them?

Quite simply you should always seek to empower your patients by encouraging them to write reviews about their experiences with you as their surgeon.

Let's break that down a little.

Reputation management is a vast and complex business sector in itself, however there are a few things you can do quickly and easily to make a real difference:

1. Postcards
   Hand out cards requesting a review and listing the sites these can be left on.

2. Emails

   As part of any post-operative care emails you send make sure you directly request reviews.

3. Invoices

   Add copy to your invoices indicating where reviews can be left.

4. Google Plus

   Set up and maintain a Google Business account where customers can easily leave appraisals of their experiences with you.

Work as hard to get reviews for your services as you do delivering them. Don't be shy in asking: the easier you make it for your patients to review your services on independent websites, the more reviews you will have.

Your online reputation is critical to your success but it is a slow burner. This is why you should be getting started today to lay the foundations for your reputation and patient numbers to grow exponentially.

Finally, I am not going to say your gift of a free book can override any negative experiences of the surgical process. But consider this: gratitude goes a long way indeed.

If your patients have felt supported throughout from their very first contact with you they are much more likely to feel disposed to leave you a review. Securing positive reviews is harder that gaining negative ones. So you have set yourself once more above your competitors because gratitude is very rarely forgotten.

Secret #4:
How You Can Use Facebook to Grow Your Prospects

"Sell-sell-sell sales methods simply do not work on social media."

Kim Garst

I'm going to state the obvious. There is a lot more you can share on Facebook than photos of cats and videos of epic fails.

I'm going to show you just why you should be using Facebook and how you can use it to promote your book, gain prospects and future-proof your practice with an exponential number of patients.

If you're looking incredulous again I'll start by outlining exactly what an opportunity Facebook represents before I show you how to grasp it with both hands.

Why Facebook?

"Nobody reads ads. People read what interests them, and sometimes it's an ad."

Howard Luck Gossage

Facebook can integrate your ads with people's lifestyles in a way no other medium has managed before. It's not only seamless: it's also incredibly wide-reaching.

Here's an amazing fact for you: Facebook now has more 'reach' than television.[iv] It allows you to reach any type of person, of any age, from any city, with any interest and at any time. What's more is it allows you to do this for a fraction of the price of television advertising.

It's time to start thinking outside the goggle-box. Your practice can finally compete for the first time with the huge clinics that spend vast amounts of money on TV, radio and newspaper advertising.

The playing field been levelled and you are in a distinct position to gain a very real competitive advantage.

You see, only 22% of businesses are actually advertising their services on Facebook.[v] When I say advertising I don't mean just creating a fan page and praying for Likes ('build it and they will come'). What I mean is actively creating advertisements.

If the opportunity is so great then where are the other 78%? It's a good question. The truth is that many businesses lack the time, resources, budget and knowledge to market themselves effectively. This is doubly true for online marketing, and trebly so for social media advertising. In fact, half of all businesses in the UK and Australia don't even have a website. [vi]

Let's just take a second to think a bit more about this. You have the chance to use a highly effective advertising platform that four out of five of your competitors are sleeping on. What's more, of the one in five who uses it, very few actually use it effectively.

I'm going to show you how to leverage a marketing channel that will place your practice in prime position to generate prospects and convert them into patients.

This is a gift horse for you, so don't look it in the mouth. Wrap your arms around it, embrace it and then run with it.

This is your chance to get ahead of the pack.

This year Facebook reached over 1.23 billion active users every month. That's a 16% increase on last year, and it's showing no signs of slowing up. People are using their desktop computers to browse Facebook. They're using their iPads. And now they're using their mobile phones. We spend more time each day browsing Facebook than we do watching TV.

This is why Facebook has replaced the television and newspapers when it comes to getting your business 'out there'. Put simply you get far greater equity for your marketing dollars with Facebook advertising.

- You get a better reach.
- You get the ability to carefully segment and precisely target your audience.

- You get much lower costs.
- You get great responses.
- And you get effective branding as Facebook keeps you in front of hundreds, thousands or even millions of people every time they check their News Feed.

This is all crucial for your practice.

By building your brand equity you gain 'first in mind' status: remember that your prospects rarely make quick overnight decisions.

By using Facebook's advertising platform you can target your marketing like never before. For example, if you were selling Mummy Makeovers in Manchester, you can target the following increasingly precise demographic:

- ✓ Mums...
- ✓ In Manchester...
- ✓ Or within 30 miles of it...
- ✓ With a new baby that is under three years old...
- ✓ Who has shown an interest in plastic surgery.

Bullseye!

Now we are on target let me explain exactly how you can reach the people you want to by using Facebook to advertise your book. Let me also reveal how this will not only supercharge your A.C.E factor, but it will also educate your prospects along the road to consultation and conversion.

How to Generate Patients Using Facebook to Promote Your Book

"Successful companies in social media function more like entertainment companies, publishers, or party planners than as traditional advertisers."

Erik Qualman

Once you have published your book one of the very best ways to get a printed copy into the hands of your prospects is to use Facebook's advertising platform.

Facebook has available an advertising method called 'Page Post Link' and it's the number one most valuable space in internet advertising that is available to you at the moment.

These ads are sometimes called News Feed ads because this is where they appear: right in the middle of your prospect's News Feed alongside updates from groups they follow and their friends' updates.

They feature a large image which is ideal for catching the wandering eye as it scrolls through the News Feed, and they are a highly effective way to promote your website and gain Likes for your fan page. And, of course, to tell people about your book.

Let's pause for breath a moment here. I am not about to tell you that understanding and implementing a Facebook advertising campaign is easy. It isn't. It takes time, skill and knowledge: this is not something I'd advise you to try at home.

What I am going to do is to make it as easy possible for you to get your focus right.

What I have done is to create a series of templates and step-by-step instructions that you can send directly to your marketing manager, or to your existing marketing agency, for implementation. My main goal here is to get you going and make sure you are going along the right tracks.

The quicker you start spreading your 'celebrity' status, the faster your appointment booking schedules will fill up.

So here it is: your step-by-step guide to creating a super-charged A.C.E factor advertising campaign.

Use it and watch the leads come in!

1. Create a fan page
   I am going to presume that your practice probably has a fan page already. If it doesn't spend a few minutes setting one up: if you need any help doing this just type 'how to create a Facebook fan page' into Google because there are plenty of easy to follow guides that are readily available.

2. Create a landing page on your website
   A landing page is where your prospect will 'land' after they click on your ad. Don't worry: I have already done all the thinking for you. I have created a template design that you can send to your web designer. All they need to do is copy and paste this design onto your website and you are ready to go.

   You can find the template by going to:
   goo.gl/c2oy42

3. Create a 'thank-you page' on your website

   A 'thank-you page' is where your website visitor arrives after they submit their information on an enquiry form. Again, I have taken care of all the technical details for you and created a template design that you can pass on to your web designer. Guess what: all they need to do is copy and paste our design onto your website and you are once more ready to go.

   You can find the template by going to:
   goo.gl/97he23

4. Create your ad

   I'm sure you are getting used to this by now so just send this to whoever is managing your Facebook advertising for you.

   You can find your ad template by going to:
   goo.gl/AZlb4h

   (You must be logged into Facebook to see this dummy ad.)

5. Choose your target audience

   Remember when creating your book, I asked you to profile your target audience? If you did your homework you are about to reap the rewards because this information is going to come in really handy when you choose the people you want to show your ads to on Facebook.

To give you an example: for one of my clients the most profitable audience has proven to be a female parent with a child under three years old, who lives within 30 kilometres of Sydney and is between 25 and 45 years old.

6. Choose a budget you are comfortable with
   Starting cautiously is fine but allocating at least £10 ($20 AUD) per day is an absolute minimum.

7. Activate your advertisement
   Sit back and watch the leads come in!

Capitalising on Facebook Ads with Direct Mail and Email Autoresponders

Did you take a look at the landing page template I created for your website?

You can find it at:
goo.gl/c2oy42

Notice how clicking the 'Send me my book' button causes a popup form to appear. This form asks for your name, email and full postal address. There is a very specific reason I have included a request for postal address details: of course, I want to send out the book in the post, but I also want to be able to send out follow up letters. These follow ups are designed to convert the now warm prospect into a consultation.

I recommend using three follow up letters that go by post and three follow up emails that are sent by your autoresponder.

The letters and emails serve the same purpose, it's just that some people prefer packages in the post and some prefer emails. For example, if you are marketing your facelift procedure to women who are over 45 years old they are more likely to open, and respond to, their post than their email. To really win at this game, you need to hit your prospects from all angles.

Here are the templates you should follow:

Email and letter #1

As soon as a prospective patient requests your book, by submitting the online form, you want to let them know that you're taking action. So you'll need to rush off confirmations to them the same day.

These will need to be written to accomplish the following:

1. Give them immediate feedback that their request has been successfully completed and registered.

2. Congratulate them on the wisdom of making the decision to request your book.

3. Provide contact information, such as an email address, should they have any questions.

4. Reinforce the benefits of the book to build their anticipation of receiving it.

Email and letter #2

The second communication in this series should be sent out after you have mailed the package and you are confident the book is in their hands. Depending on how you ship and their location the timings for this could vary, so you'll have to trial a test run to see how long delivery usually takes. Optimally, the second communication should land no more than a couple of days after the package has arrived.

The second communication will need to be written to accomplish the following:

1. Congratulate them again on being really smart for asking for the book.

2. Lay out the benefits the book offers and what they will learn by reading it.

3. Reinforce the need to go through the book, if they haven't done so already.

4. Introduce your procedure.

5. State the benefits and transformations associated with your procedure.

6. Provide a strong call to action: pick up the phone or email to find out more.

Email and letter #3

The final communication in this series should go out about three to five days after the previous.

It should be written to accomplish the following:

1. Confirm that by now they've had time to read and appreciate your book.

2. Describe why *you* can be trusted to deliver on your promises.

3. Restate the clear, massive value of your offer.

4. Close on a firm call to action once more.

Your series of emails and letters may have ended but your relationship with your prospect is not over regardless of whether they respond or not.

Your database contacts of today are your patients of tomorrow: if you are not sure what to do to make this happen you can refresh your memory on how to nurture your prospects and grow your patients by looking again at Chapter 2.

If you are ready for the next secret, however, it's time to reveal how content marketing could be taking your surgery to the next level and beyond.

Secret #5:
Generate Patients with a Supercharged Content Marketing Strategy

"Content marketing is more than a buzzword. It is the hottest trend in marketing because it is the biggest gap between what buyers want and brands produce."

Michael Brenner

A lot of agencies will tell you that you need to be blogging every week. This can often be more of a slog than a blog. What are you blogging for? Who are you blogging to? Blogging alone is simply not enough. It's just a variant on 'build it and they will come'.

Here's the rub.

When you post a blog to your site you rely on your site's visitors to find it. How many do you have? How many of these actually get to your blog? Have a look and then ask yourself why exactly you are blogging religiously once a week. Is it some form of penance?

Don't misunderstand: me there *is* a lot of value in blogs. But a post without readers is as pointless as a practice with no patients.

What you need is a way to start making your blog posts work harder, rather than wasting your time producing posts to your agency's schedule. What you need is a market for your content. It stands to reason that what you should be doing then is marketing your content, and I'm going to show you exactly how to do it.

In a nutshell: the technique I have seen work exceptionally well is writing an educational blog post and then creating a 'Promoted Post' on Facebook that is targeted towards a group of people who will be most interested in the subject matter.

Using this method it is not unusual to see more than a thousand visitors in a day actively reading your latest blog as a result. And that's worth writing a blog post for!

Let's be clear about what your 'Promoted Post' is. It's not an advert in the traditional sense. There is no sales message and no special offer. There is not even necessarily any PR intent. You are not selling: you are educating.

Why would you want to do this? Well, to truly understand the concept you are going to need to step into the shoes of your prospect.

Facebook is not AdWords. Your prospects are not in the middle of a search for the best breast augmentation surgeon in London: they are going about their daily life. But you know they are a good fit for your practice and you know that they are interested in cosmetic surgery.

So how are you going to pique their interest? How are you going to warm up these cold prospects?

Whilst they are browsing to see what their family and friends are up to they will intermittently see advertising in their News Feed. You can think of these, if you like, as ad breaks in the middle of a highly personalised TV news show. Except they are not quite so intrusive or conspicuous.

So, one of the first things you will need to do is to write a blog post with a catchy heading: something like '6 ways to...' or 'The truth about...' or 'How to ... quickly and easily'. It doesn't need to be sales driven: the important thing is you make sure it is about information people want to read about.

If you have copywriters working for you at the moment hand it over to them. If not, don't worry you can head on over to Elance (www.elance.com) or Odesk (www.odesk.com) and hire someone from there.

The real trick here is to make sure your copywriter understands that you are being useful. This is not an advert that is aiming to sell but one that is providing information.

What it needs to do is to pique interest. Make sure your agency or freelancer understands this.

Your goal is to get a prospect's attention, give them great, information and let them get to know your brand a little. You are going to save the selling for when they are 'warmed up' a little.

Let's get specific. I'm going to talk you through a few examples of ads that work, and I'm going to show you some that don't.

How do I know this?

Because these are all ads I have tested: I'll save you the learning curve!

Ads that are not going to work for cold prospects:

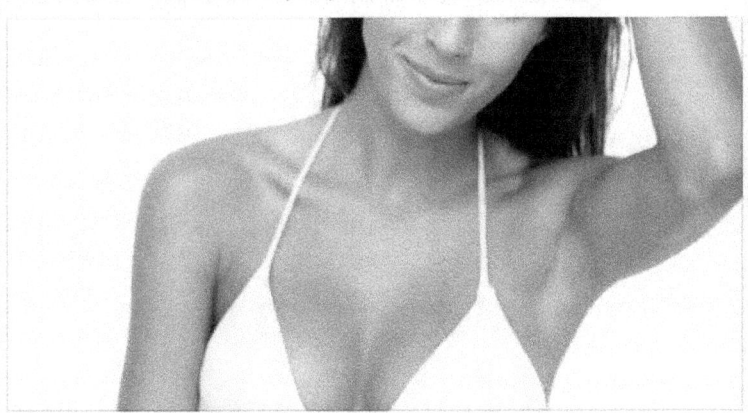

Find Out How You Can Get A Sydney Boob Job For Thailand Prices!

Sydney Breast Surgery, Thailand Prices

Breast surgery by a certified Sydney cosmetic plastic surgeon doesn't have to cost an arm and a leg, you can get it done here in Sydney for Thailand prices!

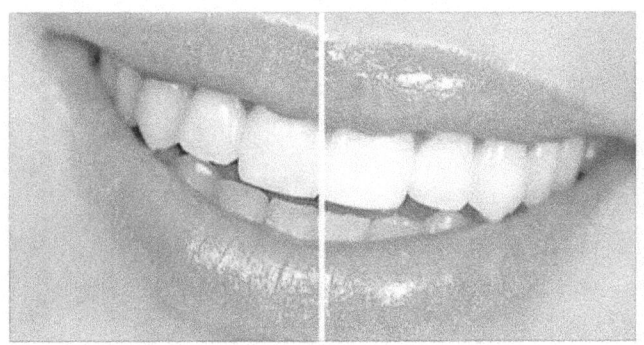

Fancy a 'celebrity smile' makeover?
Check out our discount of up to 50% on Smile Makeovers!

Up To 50% Off Smile Makeovers

Ever wanted a beautiful, pearly-white, 'Celebrity Smile'?
                    are award winning cosmetic dentists in London's most prestigious centre for dental excellence.

Ads that are prospect winners:

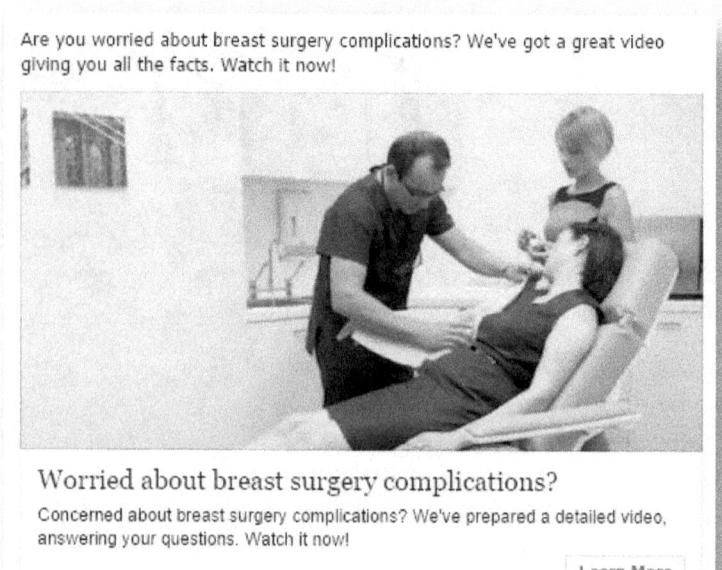

Are you worried about breast surgery complications? We've got a great video giving you all the facts. Watch it now!

Worried about breast surgery complications?

Concerned about breast surgery complications? We've prepared a detailed video, answering your questions. Watch it now!

Learn More

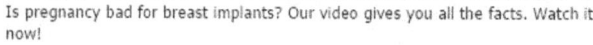

Is pregnancy bad for breast implants? Our video gives you all the facts. Watch it now!

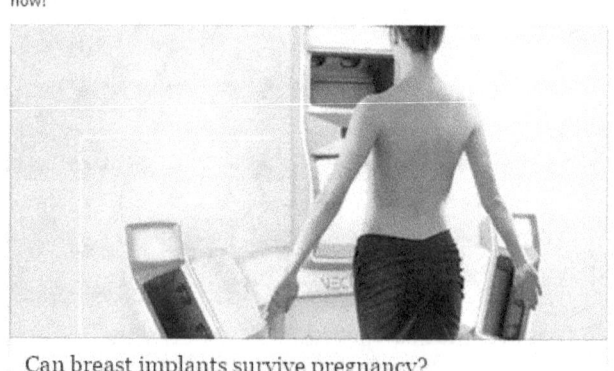

Can breast implants survive pregnancy?

What happens to breast implants during pregnancy? We've prepared a detailed video, answering your questions. Watch it now!

Learn More

Do you see the difference?

The first two are selling, and the second two are educating. The irony is that it is the informative and useful ads, rather than the offer driven sales monsters, that will achieve your surgery's goals of growing your prospective patients.

But, you might ask, how can I turn these educational ads into patients?

Drumroll, please...

...I'm going to get a smidgen technical here...

...By using Facebook's 'Website Custom Audience (WCA)' facility...

...Cymbal crash!

Bear with me: I'll make this as painless as possible.

WCA is Facebook's fancy version of remarketing. It means that any person who visits your website by clicking on your educational ad, can be tagged and added to a series of your 'lists', depending on what content they are reading.

These lists could, for example, be split up into procedure types. You can call on your lists at any time and show a more sales-oriented 'book a consultation' ad to only these people.

It is genius really:

- Educate the prospect.
- Warm them up.
- Then hit them with a 'book a consultation' ad.

They trust you. They appreciate that you know what you are talking about.

They have learnt from you. You are no longer a pushy practice selling but a surgery your prospect might well consider when the time is right.

Now do you understand why you are creating blog posts and advertising them on Facebook?

Now are the benefits of educational ads making more sense?

To summarise:

1. Facebook is not Google.
2. Your prospects are often very early in their decision making process.
3. You need to warm them up first before you sell to them!

But it's not just Facebook that can turn prospects into patients through remarketing.

Remarketing is far too powerful a tool to leave to just one platform: that is why my next secret is going to be telling you more about it as a tactic and trying to convince you that your budget for it should be as much as you can spare.

No-one likes to hear that.

But you will find it will all come back to you.

And the rest!

Secret #6:
Use Remarketing to Convert Interest into Action

"Content is anything that adds value to the reader's life."

Avinash Kaushik

I love the quote that opens this chapter.

"Content is anything that adds value to the reader's life."

It's from a key person at Google and I understand it to say that effective advertising is not an intrusion or an interruption. It is an enhancement: it adds value by being in the right place at the right time with an interesting message.

I thought of this the other day when I was looking to go on holiday. I'd been searching for a break away online, only to find that one of the operator's websites seemed to appear enticingly on several websites as an advert a couple of days later whilst I was online working for a client.

The ad promised more information about the sandy beach resorts I had been looking at and even made a rather compelling offer. I clicked on the ad eventually and the site was informative and the offer seductive. I made the booking.

The holiday was great!

This advertising that seems to follow you after you have visited a site is called remarketing. It's an effective tactic as my booking attests. What remarketing allows you to do is to convert initial interest into action by keeping you front of mind.

Remarketing ensures that a route back to your site is always present. The easier you make it to find out more or make that enquiry the more prospects become patients.

Here is the problem that remarketing so elegantly solves. You invest in online marketing to drive prospects to your website. You may use display advertising, you may use pay per click or you may make a monthly spend on optimising your site for the search engines. It doesn't matter: the point is that each visitor costs you money. If each visit represents an investment it's only natural that you should be trying to make the most of your spend.

Yet, for most of cosmetic surgery clients, approximately 2% of their visitors get in touch via phone or email.

Two in every hundred! That is a pittance!

Remarketing is a tool designed to help you reach the 98% who will probably otherwise just vanish into the ether.

That is a blessing!

Remarketing is so effective because it focuses your advertising spend on people who are already familiar with your brand and have recently demonstrated interest. That's why most surgeons who use it see a higher ROI than they do from most other digital channels.

So remarketing repays your spend in two ways. First, it gives you a great return through strong results. Second, it gives you the chance to maximise on your other investments to drive visits.

Here's how the virtuous remarketing circle works as it transforms potential into profit:

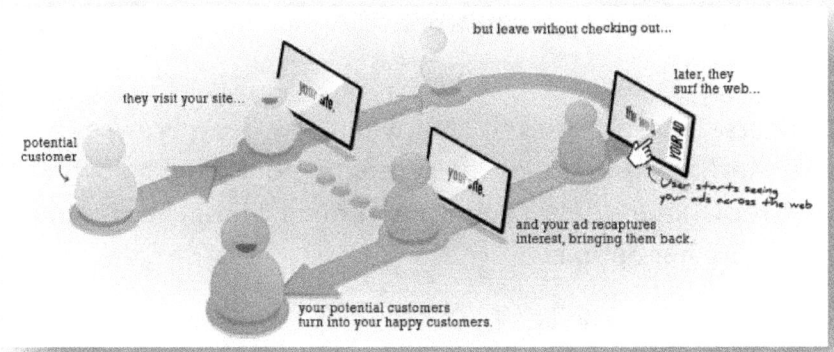

Just to make sure you grasp this enormous opportunity fully I'm going to give you a more concrete example of its magic at work.

Meet Alexis.

She is a self-proclaimed '30 something' mother of two.

Now that the kids are in their schools, Alexis is considering abdominoplasty: it's time to treat herself.

The house is quiet at 4pm on a Wednesday afternoon when Alexis stumbles upon your website through a well-placed pay per click ad on Google.

Alexis is interested.

She is about to fill out the contact form when the kids (Evie and Finn) bounce through the front door and she distractedly bounces off your site.

Should we wave bye to Alexis or could you try and restart what she had to finish?

Through remarketing the next time Alexis surfs, during a quiet moment at home, your banner ads can show up on many websites around the internet: shopping channels, make-up retailers, TV listings, Facebook, news sites.

Your brand will be back in front of Alexis allowing her to get back in touch.

Of course, it's just as likely that when, say, Jane browses your site she has no intention of getting in touch right now. Still your remarketing keeps you front of mind whilst she continues to explore her options.

We all love the familiar.

We trust it.

Remarketing helps you build trust through familiarity. And it keeps you always close at hand.

Remarketing is an extremely powerful tool. If your agency is not using it for your benefit don't hesitate to ask them why. If they can't answer you may want to reconsider your relationship with them.

The bottom line is that these ads costs very little compared to their ROI.

The top tip is to spend as much as you can on remarketing!

Conversion Begins at Home

"Sometimes the questions are complicated and the answers are simple."

Dr. Seuss

We are now almost there.

You have six secrets that will skyrocket your surgical practice's marketing.

Each secret is in itself an innovative, creative response to a complex problem that you have been battling with for your practice.

Each secret unlocks another way to find prospects, capture their interest, get their details and nurture them.

Albert Einstein, a man who knew a lot about both creativity and intelligence, once said that "creativity is intelligence having fun."

It's true: intelligence is applying creative solutions to problems that are unique, perhaps even slightly off the wall.

I've been doing this with cosmetic surgeons for many years now, and I still find it fun. I'm a competitive guy so fun for me is beating the field, streaking away and slamming the ball in the basket.

Fun for me is winning.

But there are still a few seconds left on the clock before the game ends, and there is still an opportunity to get into another huddle and take a time-out.

Let's do it because I have one more secret I need to give to you that's going to really boost your game to the next level.

What could really tip the scales in your favour is to take that 2% conversion rate that you probably have for first-time visitors and increase it.

Believe me just taking it from 2% to 3% makes a big difference (after all it's a 50% increase).

To do this we need to focus on conversion.

We need to furnish you with a powerful procedure page that can provide that final clear call to action to every visit you have.

I'm going to next lay bare the anatomy of just such a page for you.

And then it will truly be game over for the competition.

Let's do this!

Secret #7:
The Perfect Procedure Page

"If content is king, then conversion is queen."

John Munsell

Agencies love to discuss the metrics that drive visitors to your site. Given the chance most will happily while away the day explaining tactics to improve these.

Let's tick a few of these off to keep them happy:

- ✓ CTR (Clickthrough rate)
- ✓ CPC (Cost per click)
- ✓ CPM (Cost per thousand impressions)
- ✓ Quality Score
- ✓ Average Position

These are all important metrics, so much so that you could realistically dribble on about them all day, but the gains made from improving on any of the above are miniscule compared to the improvements you can gain from having a website that impresses, is laid out well, is mobile friendly and, as a result, converts.

Think of it this way: if you have a website that converts better than your competitors, you can pay more for your advertising and still win.

Or this way: let's say you are receiving only half of your competitor's visitors, yet you are getting double their patients. Who is marketing effectively?

Conversion is a pretty cool tactic and here is how you can own it.

Don't worry I haven't forgotten you are a plastic surgeon. It's not your job to split test your site to improve conversion rates or to spend your time making incremental design and copy changes to your key pages. (To be honest your marketing agency should be already doing this for you. They are, aren't they?)

I'm going to keep this simple because it's important you understand it completely and carry it out. After all, it is in your interests to grow your own practice.

The problem is that if you leave this to your web designer the job will not get done. Designers know how to make things pretty, but very few have the foggiest about turning cold visits into consultations. And, if you listen carefully, somewhere in the background your agency is probably still extolling the virtues of reducing lost impression share. Let's leave them to it, shall we?

I'm going to provide you with a simple check list that will ensure your website ticks all the conversion boxes. Make sure you follow this and you will see your website convert to its full potential.

1. Is your website responsive (or mobile-friendly)?

A comScore report recently revealed that smartphones and tablets now account for 60% of all online traffic (up from 50% a year ago).[vii]

If your site is not designed to display on a mobile or tablet you are fighting a losing battle from the get go. The majority of your visitors are unlikely to get beyond its landing page let alone carry out any meaningful research or actions. Spend a little bit of money converting your site as soon as you can.

2. Do you have separate 'landing pages' for different types of visitors?

We still see too many surgeons sending website traffic to their home page alone.

What's wrong with this?

Well, let's assume someone is looking for 'chin augmentation'. On one site they land on a page that talks about the procedure, the whole procedure and nothing but the procedure. On another they arrive at a generic home page that more likely than not features mainly breast augmentation information. Which site would you guess gets the most enquiries?

You need to create a new web page for each procedure, and I'll show you just how to do this next.

You need to make sure that these pages are being used as the landing pages for the relevant ads you pay for, or you risk severely losing your ability to gain a good return on your investments.

3. Are your landing pages designed to effectively convert visitors into prospects?

If this all sounds a bit technical read on to find out just how simple this actually is to do. You'll wonder why you haven't done it.

- The first thing is you need to make it as easy as possible to get in contact. You didn't enter this business to accrue secret admirers from afar did you?

  Each page should offer a clear and direct way for people to get in touch via email without having to go to another page to do this.

Your phone number should always be visible and, as much as 60% of your visitors could be using a mobile device, it must be designed so it can be clicked on to contact you.

- You should use your 'sidebar' to promote your special offers.

- You should get a good copywriter who knows how to write what your visitors want to hear!

That's it.

It's not that there isn't more you could do, it's just that most cosmetic surgery sites fail to get these basics right. If you can do just this you will see the results very quickly.

The follow page has a good example of a procedure page that is built to convert:

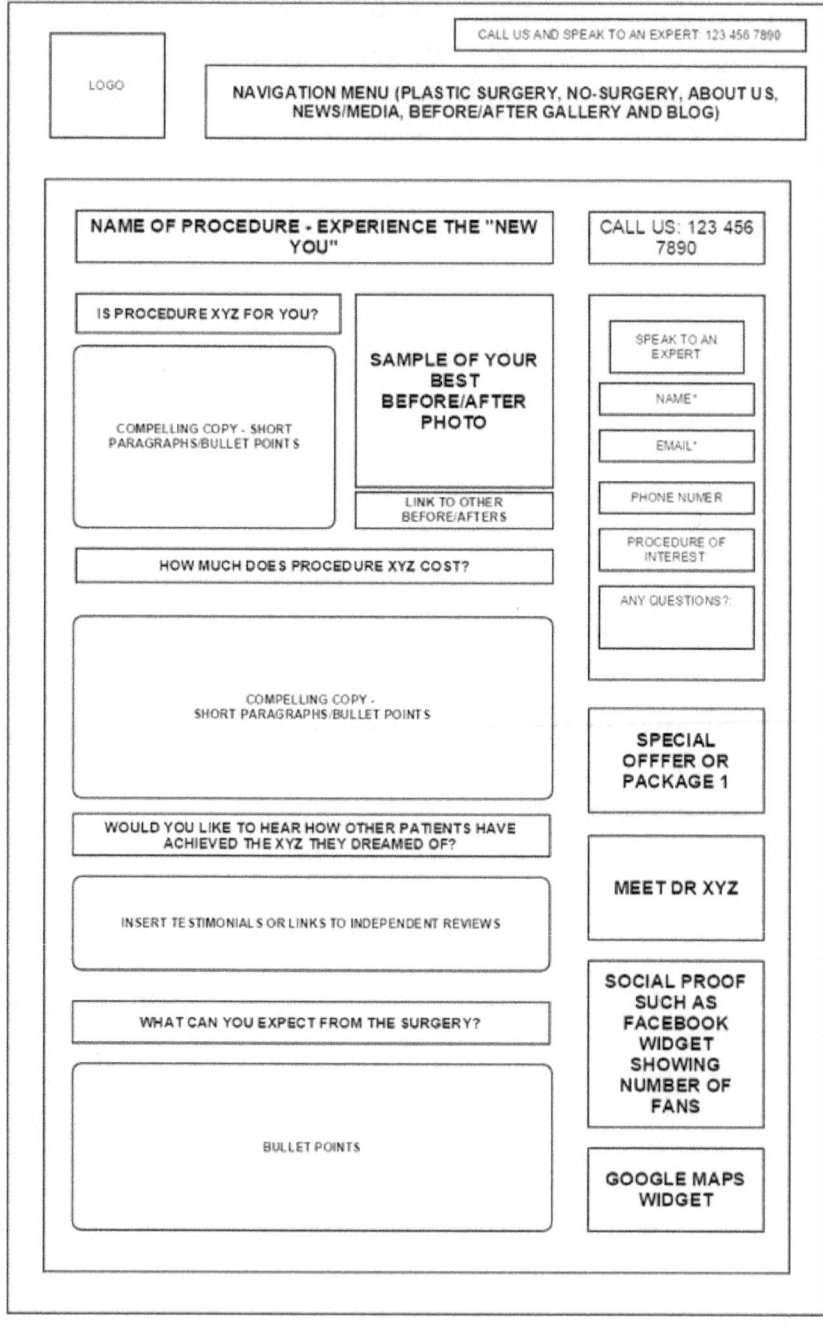

As you can see it's not rocket science.

But it works.

And it works like a dream.

Your website's ability to convert is way too important to be left in the hands of those whose concerns are elsewhere. Take control by clearly briefing your agency or designer what your priorities actually are.

Do it today because you will start benefitting from your changes tomorrow.

Conclusion:
Playing the Joker

"Each player must accept the cards life deals him or her: but once they are in hand, he or she alone must decide how to play the cards in order to win the game."

Voltaire

The cards are in your hand: you must decide how to play them.

As a marketing strategy for a cosmetic surgeon writing a book may seem like the Joker in the pack, but you can use it to rewrite the rules. And, of course, let's not forget that the Joker can sometimes be the highest trump card there is.

I have shown you the secrets that I have used to unleash the full power of patient generation. It starts with gaining the A.C.E factor by becoming an author. I have then shown you how you can leverage your newfound powers to find prospects, command their attention, capture their details, nurture their trust and convert them into patients and ambassadors for your practice.

You now have a whole armoury of tactics, tips and templates to make a game plan, up your game and change the game forever.

For the last few years I have helped cosmetic surgery practices just like yours stop struggling to achieve incremental growth and start realising exponential increases. There's no longer any need to ask me how I did it: it's all in this book.

It's your turn now.

What you have read is a guide to how success lies in your hands. And you can create it all largely on your own.

Flexx Digital (www.flexxdigital.com) is the name of my marketing agency that specialises in working with the cosmetic surgery industry in the UK and Australia. We are always here to help if you need us or just want to smooth out any wrinkles. We've been there, seen that and achieved it many times before, yet it still excites us as if it were the first time.

It's your play now.

Game on.

An Unexpected Bonus

"Now this is not the end. It is not even the beginning of the end. But it is, perhaps, the end of the beginning."

Winston Churchill

What are you waiting for?

You have all you need to unleash the full potential of patient generation. Honestly.

If you need help let's talk.

+44 1273 25 2142

+61 2 8091 6982

As you are still reading I can let you in on a bonus secret.

One of the biggest impediments to getting the big things done is all those little things that get in your way. I've learnt from many surgeries how this can become a real problem. Then again, from just a few I've picked up some great ways to clear the crap out of your practice and out of everyone's hair.

So now you'll be able to breathe again and get on with the things that matter.

Like writing that book...

Bonus Secret:
How to Outsource the Crap in Your Practice

"The key is not to prioritize what's on your schedule, but to schedule your priorities."

Stephen Covey

The truth may hurt a little, but I have to say it.

Doctors are not usually great businessmen.

Just because you are skilled in surgery does not mean you also have an in-depth understanding of how to build a successful business.

The reality is, knowing how to be a doctor has very little to do with knowing how to market and run a practice.

If you are you feeling overworked and like you are juggling too many tasks then you will enjoy this short and succinct tutorial. It will reveal how you can systematically outsource all the crap on your 'to do list' with the help of high-quality virtual assistants.

I call them VAs for short.

But you could call them lifesavers.

The 'One Thing'...

"Success demands singleness of purpose. You need to be doing fewer things for more effect instead of doing more things with side effects."

Gary Keller

The first time I ever heard of 'the one thing' was in a book whose title was the same. 'The One Thing' is written by Gary Keller and I cannot recommend it enough.

In fact, I just *can't stop* recommending it.

If you ever feel that you need to get things done then this book will help you to:

- Cut through the clutter.
- Achieve better results in less time.
- Build momentum toward your goal.
- Dial down the stress.
- Overcome that overwhelmed feeling.
- Stay on track.
- Master what matters to you.

Extraordinary results happen only when you are able to focus and concentrate on what's most important to you. For surgeons and medical professionals what is truly important is to be recognised as the best there is for your chosen procedure.

But to be the best you are going to need to find ways to deal with the crap that comes with being a surgeon in a busy practice.

What Gary Keller taught me is that "multitasking is a lie".

He advises you to forget trying to do it. It just doesn't work.

The only thing that trying to multitask achieves is to dilute your focus and your results.

It is the single-minded that achieve great results.

In our frantic scramble to be and do everything we end up as and with nothing. As we race from one little thing to the next we leave behind the Big Thing that we actually should be achieving.

Unless we can clear the crap the Big Thing will never even get completed, let alone successfully completed.

This simple truth changed my life.

And it is the 'one thing' that could be making a profound impact on you reaching your goals too.

I listen to my books, rather than read them. Using Amazon's Audible service (www.audible.co.uk) you can get a free trial for a month here in the UK. If you haven't done so already, plug your smartphone in with a set of headphones and give Gary Keller's book a go.

You can find it here:

http://goo.gl/MGz498

Applying the 'One Thing' Theory

"Be like a postage stamp — stick to one thing until you get there."

Josh Billings

It's frustrating isn't it?

So often you *know* exactly what needs to done to double your business. And then the daily barrage of emails, texts, tweets, messages and meetings distract you and the stress of it all prevents anything truly constructive from getting done.

The problem is that all these commitments are just bottlenecks that prevent you from doing the 'one thing' that is actually going to have the biggest impact.

This is why you need 'outsourcers' to remove your bottlenecks: once these are gone you'll be free to work on making your business expand and grow like crazy.

Let's list those things that create bottlenecks right now. You know, the things that collectively prevent you achieving your goals and stunt the growth of your practice.

It's going to take some simple maths to define the issues.

If you want to earn, say, £1 million ($2 million AUD) each year, then any internal task where the investment is £500 ($1,000 AUD) an hour or less should be outsourced.

That means you should not be doing your own invoices. It means you should not be editing your own photos or videos. It means a lot of you daily, weekly or monthly tasks should barely touch your desk.

Here is a list of typical bottlenecks experienced by most small and medium businesses:

- Accounts
- Scheduling meetings
- Data entry
- Social media updates
- Direct mail
- Graphic design for flyers and advertising
- General paperwork
- Invoices
- Video production
- Research
- Blog writing
- Transcription
- Patient Support

The list could go on and on: I'm sure you can fill in the rest. In fact, I'm going to suggest you do just that in a moment.

What if you could remove these bottlenecks?

What if there was a way to take a larger view of your business and systematically began removing every single one of them?

What would happen to your stress levels, your effectiveness, your business, your number of new patients and your income?

'What if' is for dreamers: it's time to make it happen.

Outsourcing Your Way Around Bottlenecks

I had a big problem within my own business.

It had expanded like crazy over the last three years. Not to brag but I was driving £1 million (or $2 million AUD) worth of paid traffic to my clients' sites, managing their ad accounts, making changes to my own website, hiring people, writing copy, doing our own marketing, getting banners designed for campaigns and acting as the single point of contact for 'support' questions!

It probably sounds familiar, right?

The painful truth is that, whilst I soldiered on thinking I was doing the right thing, there just was never time for the 'one thing' that my business actually needed: to move up to the next level.

I just wasn't able to find the time to take it there.

And then I read 'The One Thing'.

I committed immediately to hiring top quality, skilled 'virtual assistants' (VAs) who could do all the stuff which was bogging me down.

Within weeks I had two VAs doing everything I hated doing. Invoicing, support tickets, bookkeeping and research: the lot.

I could breathe.

I could think.

I started to act.

And my business has entered the nest level.

Where You Can Find Amazing Virtual Assistants *Today*

Why hire a full-time *local* employee when, in most cases, all that you need is a full-time virtual assistant?

A VA is someone who works remotely and can handle numerous assorted tasks for you. They cost between £3-500 ($6-900 AUD) a month and they will take care of all those little things that stop you working on that Big Thing.

A quick side note on hiring 'part-time' VAs.

Part-time hires is not something that I often do. I work in a pretty structured way and can usually predict what I need in advance.

The true value I'm talking about here comes from full-time assistance.

For the occasional 'one and done' project there are two sites I have mentioned before that can be relied on for part-time VAs: Elance.com and Odesk.com.

But let's get back to the meat in this sandwich.

When it comes to full-time VAs I am going to have to issue a word of warning. For a variety of reasons I have found hiring workers based in India to be a complete nightmare. I have never had a single hire from India pan out on an ongoing basis. The attention to detail just hasn't been there for me and that means I'm back in bottleneck city again.

I don't doubt there are others who have had a different experience entirely: for me, having hired dozens of VAs in India, I won't be doing it again.

I have had the best experience hiring people from within the Philippines. For a start Filipinos are more fluent in English compared to other countries like India and China. More than this, however, is the fact that I have found Filipino VAs to be flexible, smart, competent and reliable.

If I were to be completely honest with you I have found that, in many cases, Filipino VAs are actually much better than me at doing the tasks.

So, here is what you need to do to rid your business of bottlenecks and start concentrating on that one Big Thing again.

1. Get away from the office for the morning.

2. Go to your local coffee shop where you know you won't be bothered.

3. Switch off the mobile.

4. And breathe.

5. Make a list of all the bottlenecks that are holding you back from doubling your practice.

6. Look at your list.

7. Commit yourself to systematically eliminating each bottleneck.

8. Now go and hire a VA or a team of VAs.

9. Congratulations: get out there and get those results.

There are only two sites I use for hiring my VAs:

Virtual Staff Finder (www.virtualstafffinder.com/)

Online Jobs (www.onlinejobs.ph/)

But it's not a matter of just pick and click. Like any hire you will need to go through a screening process to ensure you are hiring only the most competent of applicants. To do this I have developed a survey form that I am happy to share with you.

You can find it here:

goo.gl/zl4DSh

Hiring VAs couldn't be easier. Nor could it be more effective for the health of your business (or your own mental health to come to that).

Visit the sites, register and start running ads.

My final parting tip to you: if you need to explain things quickly use 'Jing Project' to grab images from your screen and quickly mark them up with text.

You can find it at:

www.techsmith.com/jing.html

And with that I'm done.

Let me know how you get on.

Notes

Rather than clutter up this book with sources and references I include any extra information you may need here. I have used the Google URL shortener to make life easier for you.

---

[i] http://goo.gl/EyKxb4
This quote comes from Dan's excellent website (http://gkic.com) where you can learn more about his approach to marketing.
[ii] http://goo.gl/vt4ciJ
From the ASPS website (www.plasticsurgery.org.au).
[iii] http://goo.gl/wDM4mV
From the CAP website (www.cap.org.uk).
[iv] http://goo.gl/d56nEr
[v] http://goo.gl/PWyDlg
[vi] http://goo.gl/Viwgvw
[vii] http://goo.gl/joso9V

www.ingramcontent.com/pod-product-compliance
Lightning Source LLC
Chambersburg PA
CBHW051809170526
45167CB00005B/1948